THIS JOURNAL BELONGS TO:

_____

_____

_____

i am f*cking radiant

A SELF-CARE JOURNAL TO HELP YOU DITCH THE FACE MASKS, QUIT THE BULLSH*T, AND ACTUALLY FEEL F*CKING BETTER

D. A. SARAC

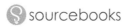

Copyright © 2020 by Sourcebooks
Cover and internal design © 2020 by Sourcebooks
Cover and internal design by Christine Webster
Cover and internal illustrations by Christine Webster

Sourcebooks and the colophon are registered trademarks of Sourcebooks.

Published by Sourcebooks
P.O. Box 4410, Naperville, Illinois 60567–4410
(630) 961-3900
sourcebooks.com

Printed and bound in Singapore.
OGP 10 9 8 7 6 5 4 3 2 1

AH, SELF-CARE...

Yoga classes, green juice, bubble baths, face goop.

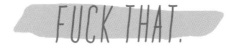

The new self-care is all about taking care of yourself in whatever way you need to feel good. Whatever your paycheck or location, your identity, social class, race, gender—self-care belongs to YOU.

Self-care is not about brands, fads, or going broke. It's about identifying your core values and making the time to nurture them. It's building a life day to day that you don't need to retreat from. It's about discovering the fantastic things about you and fueling that pure awesome energy. It's feeling all the feelings; it's standing up and making change. It's recognizing that investing in yourself is not a selfish act.

Let's first explore the fine art of self-care, then we'll learn new ways to bring out the badass in you and load up your tool belt to take charge of your own self-care! So, get out your sunglasses and prepare to be fucking RADIANT!

WHO
the fuck
DECIDED SELF-CARE
HAS TO LOOK LIKE A
skinny woman
WEARING A
$40 FACE MASK?

REDEFINING THE SELF-CARE MOVEMENT

Self-care has been branded for the skinny Instagram influencers doing all the yoga in their $150 athleisure while drinking their green juices and touting their skincare routine. And guess what? That's fucking bullshit. Self-care is for all of us—it's for the busy bitches, the stressed-out queens, the people who are doing it all and just need a minute for themselves. It's for the anxiety-ridden, the wellness-challenged, the readers who need a break to focus on their own mental health. It's for everyone. Repeat after me: SELF-CARE IS FOR FUCKING EVERYBODY.

Self-care isn't about expensive brands, spending money, or instagramming your poke bowl. It's about refocusing on yourself and listening to your mental and emotional needs. Which is why it's time to redefine self-care. To pull the focus back on what (and who) is most important.

So why is our culture suddenly making self-care a BFD (big fucking deal)? List a few reasons why you think there is a need for seven fucking gazillion books and products out there on self-care.

- help with mental illness
- for fun
- because why not
- idk

How have you viewed self-care in the past?
What does that phrase mean to you?

I have always looked at it as doing the things you love or have been wanting to do and escaping reality for a while. To me self-care means doing what makes you happy.

BUILD SOME
definition

25LB

50LB

Check off the phrases that define self-care for you.

- [x] Slow breathing in times of stress.
- [ ] Wearing my favorite shirt two days in a row. Just because.
- [ ] IDC what you say: face masks make me feel good as hell.
- [x] Not always answering texts.
- [ ] Going for a mindful walk.
- [x] Saying no to plans when I'm overwhelmed.
- [x] OH GOD A NAP, YES.
- [ ] Pizza delivery for dinner because I don't need to cook every goddamn day.
- [x] Taking my makeup off at the end of the night.
- [x] A night out on the town.
- [ ] Reading an entire book.
- [ ] Incorporating some form of joyful movement into my life.
- [ ] Soaking in the tub while reading a cozy mystery.
- [ ] Meditation or quiet time.
- [ ] A solid exercise routine that gives me the confidence to slay.
- [ ] Scented candles in every room.
- [x] ~~Cocktails~~ with my best friends.
- [x] ~~A glass of wine and~~ a Netflix special.
- [ ] Athleisure. All damn day.
- [ ] Sweating in a yoga studio.
- [ ] Eating at my favorite restaurant, just because.
- [x] Did you say skincare routine?
- [ ] Social media detox.
- [ ] Rearranging my bookshelf. Hey, don't judge.
- [x] Add. To. Fuckin'. Cart.

I'm only 14 ♡? (handwritten)

How have you practiced self-care in the past? Why do you think you need to focus on your own self-care now?

I usually go shopping and take care of my skin.

I think I need self-care because a lot has been going on and I'm super stressed.

A good night's sleep is necessary to get you through those fucking Mondays (or Tuesdays, Wednesdays, Thursdays, Fridays). What is your sleep routine like?

Sometimes I fall asleep around 8-9 and wake up around 7 and sometimes I stay up until like 12-1 and wake up around 7.

it's NEVER consistant

CATCH THE
motherfucking
Z'S

Circle which best describes your bedtime sleep habits.

A. I start my sleep ritual at the same time every night.
B. I start my sleep ritual at the same hour most of the week. Who am I kidding? At least it's dark outside.
C. *(circled)* What the fuck is a sleep ritual?

A. Once I finish my bedtime routine, I'm calm and on my pillow ready for sleep.
B. I finish my routine, but I still have a few things to take care of before actually lying down.
C. What the fuck is a bedtime routine?
D. *(circled)* Stay up on my phone

A. I'm able to sleep through the night and wake up refreshed.
B. *(circled)* With all those thoughts swimming around, it sometimes takes me a while to put the cell phone out of reach and finally get to sleep.
C. *(circled)* What the fuck is sleep?

Answers
If you picked A's, you're beyond fucking awesome.
If you picked B's, you're on the right track but can up your game.
If you picked even one C, girl, we got a shitload of work to do.

Write down what you are going to do to fix that nighttime routine and get your ass to sleep at a decent hour.

Start doing skin care at a decent time and put my phone away when I need to sleep.

Oh look. You've got the afternoon off. (It's about fucking time.)
Describe your ideal afternoon of uninterrupted self-care.

_____

_____

_____

_____

_____

Now imagine if you had twenty-four glorious hours of
self-care, all expenses paid. What's that look like?

_____

_____

_____

_____

_____

What about a week of pure, unending self-care?
What would you be doing?

HERE'S THE
scoop

Okay, so now you've got the whole day free. Silently read the first column, then shout (and I do mean fucking shout) out the new you column.

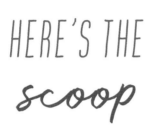

OLD ME

I have too many chores today.
I have too many errands today.
I need to answer all this email.

NEW ME

Fuck chores. I'm making a sundae.
Fuck errands. I'm making a sundae.
Fuck email. I'm making a sundae.

YOU GET THE
idea

List three of your excuses for not practicing self-care, then fix it with your new attitude.

OLD ME

1 _____

2 _____

3 _____

NEW ME

1 _____

2 _____

3 _____

List a few routines you've tried that just don't work for you.

_____

_____

_____

_____

_____

Now throw those damn things away. Let's find out what does work for you.

What's one self-care routine you've heard about but were a little embarrassed to try. Oh c'mon, spill!

_____

_____

_____

_____

Describe your ideal outfit that will make you feel amazing. Is it formal? Casual? Cosplay?

What are a couple of aromas that always make you feel better?

_____

_____

_____

I bet you did something nice for yourself this week that you can
develop into a regular self-care routine. What was it?

_____

_____

_____

_____

_____

_____

_____

_____

_____

_____

_____

_____

Did you miss a chance during the week to take care of yourself? Describe the situation.

_____

What did you do instead?

_____

You've finally found an hour to be good to yourself.
What is the one goddamn thing that always messes that up?

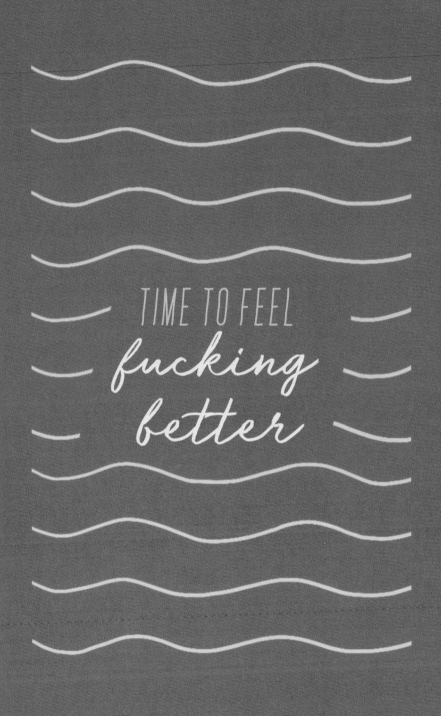

TIME TO FEEL
fucking
better

Say you're exhausted and drowsy at work. And it's only two in the afternoon. Come up with a solution to refresh yourself that doesn't include coffee or donuts. (I know. Shocking.)

_____

_____

_____

_____

_____

_____

_____

_____

_____

_____

_____

_____

Thinking back over this past week, when could you have stopped what you were doing and said "Nope, I don't give a shit"?

What's your favorite song to belt out that makes you feel so damn good?

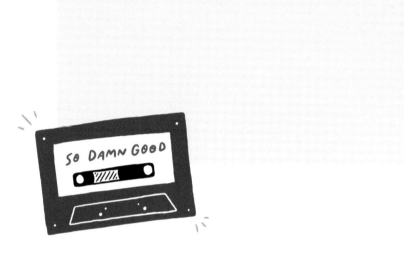

What's one favorite food item you can add to your regular grocery list to always have handy for those messed-up, no-good, goddamn horrible days?

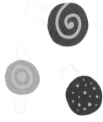

Now that we have an idea what self-care can look like, check off where your starting point is.

☐ I did self-care a few years ago.

☐ I might have lit a candle last year.

☐ There was some wine and I think a movie a few months back.

☐ Every two months I try to take a day off.

☐ I'm at the damn gym once or twice a week.

☐ Once a week is bubble-bath night. Keep out.

☐ Every weekend I unwind with friends and fun.

☐ At least three days a week. Really.

☐ Every fucking day. I am the queen of self-care.

Make a promise to incorporate one self-care routine to start off your day. Describe it here.

THE

royal

treatment

You think you're the queen of self-care yet?
Select True or False, then see how you do.

T F I have new ideas to use for this month's self-care.

T F I scheduled one day a week for self-care.

T F I will not answer every goddamn text as soon as
I hear the swoosh.

T F I know three ways to incorporate movement into my day.

T F I can focus on my breathing no matter how large the
crowd size.

T F I told my house/roommate I needed some quiet time
to get work done.

T F I went outside after a rain and just breathed in the
freshness.

T F I went to the store and just inhaled all the candles in
the home furnishings aisle and even bought one.

T F I tried a few incense sticks, then realized I was
supposed to light only one at a time.

T F I can balance my damn chakras in the morning
even if I'm late for work.

Count up all the True responses.

Five or more: You are indeed the Queen. We bow to you.
Four: Princess. Don't worry, you still get to wear the crown.
Three: Duchess. That's okay. You're in line.
Two: Lady. Hey, at least you'll be invited to tea.
One: Peasantry. No tea, no crown. But you can try again.
Zero: Do this entire journal three times. At least.

RECOGNIZE THAT
badass bitch
IN YOU.

IT'S ALL ABOUT THE SELF-LOVE

Self-care starts when we look inward and take stock of our lives. Who are we? What do we love about ourselves? Where are our roadblocks and what do we ultimately want to accomplish? When was the last time we felt confident, brave, strong?

Take a good, long look in the mirror and realize that there's a badass staring back at you. Someone who will take no prisoners, who can conquer the world, and get all the shit done! That person deserves to be treated with a helluva lot of respect, and it's time to do just that. Polish up that crown, because you're about to be wearing it all damn day.

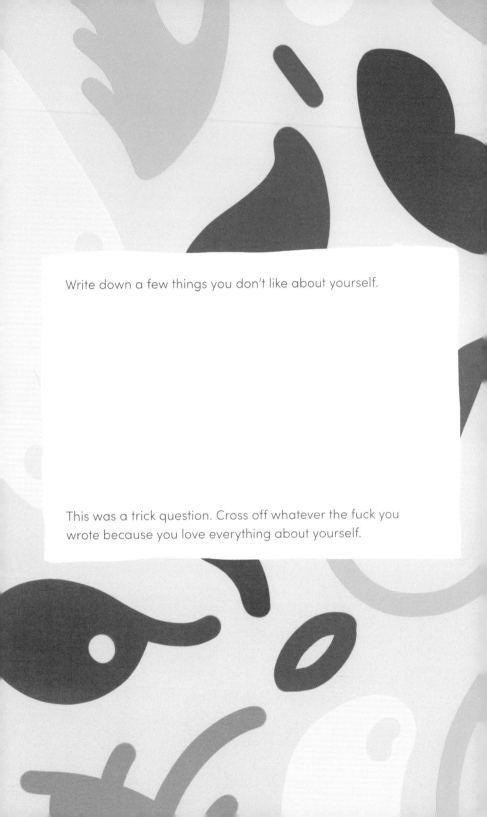

Write down a few things you don't like about yourself.

This was a trick question. Cross off whatever the fuck you wrote because you love everything about yourself.

Write down a few of your traits you are proud of.
Do not leave this page blank.

Now write down what you think others love about you.
There had better be words all over this goddamn page.

_____

_____

_____

_____

_____

_____

_____

_____

_____

_____

_____

_____

_____

_____

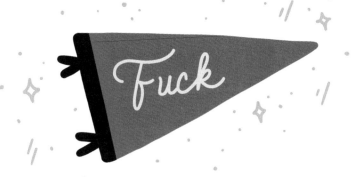

Write down a phrase someone said to you recently that pissed you off.

_____

_____

_____

_____

Now write down what you wish you could have said to that person. Let the curse words fly, girl!

_____

_____

_____

_____

_____

_____

What's one characteristic of your best friend that you truly admire? Why?

Describe the most recent time you felt strong enough to handle every fucking thing.

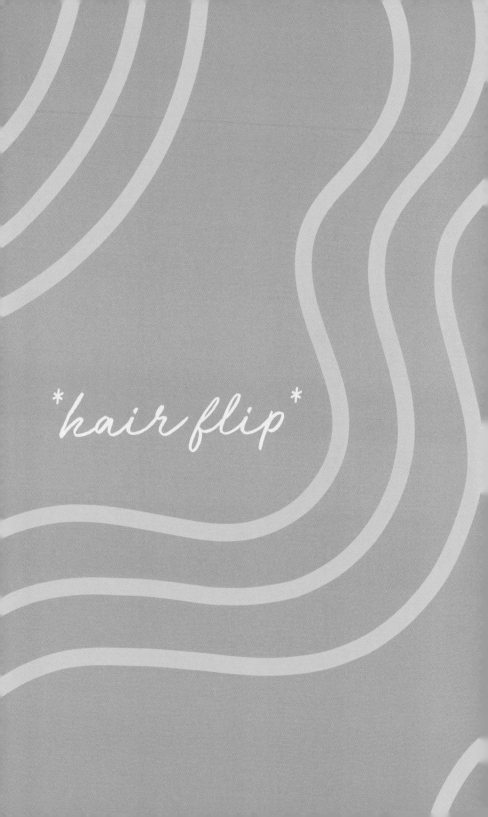

hair flip

Check off any of these badass traits you possess:

- I can pass up a group selling Girl Scout cookies. I said *can*, not will.
- That's right. I binge-watched the entire series last night.
- When a friend comes over, I can slide laundry under the couch, shove papers behind the TV, spray the air, and get the coffee brewing—all before the third knock.
- Master chef? Oh yes, that's me. The person who sautéed a vegetable today.
- I pet all the dogs. ALL of them.
- I don't have time for fucking office drama.
- I actually drank my eight glasses of water today.
- I have a kickass karaoke routine that brings a room to tears.
- I can return the online purchase I know I'm not going to use.
- I always put my grocery cart away in the parking lot.
- In traffic I let others merge ahead of me because I am that good of a person.
- I say "I'm not your goddamn doormat" out loud.
- Even on my IDGAF days, my manicure is on point.
- I can identify a coffee's country of origin by scent alone.
- I ignore an unknown caller ID and look the other way until the ringing stops.
- I get the damn flash drive into the port in one try.

What celebrity epitomizes badassery? Why?

When was the last time you felt like an absolute stunning
ball of radiance?

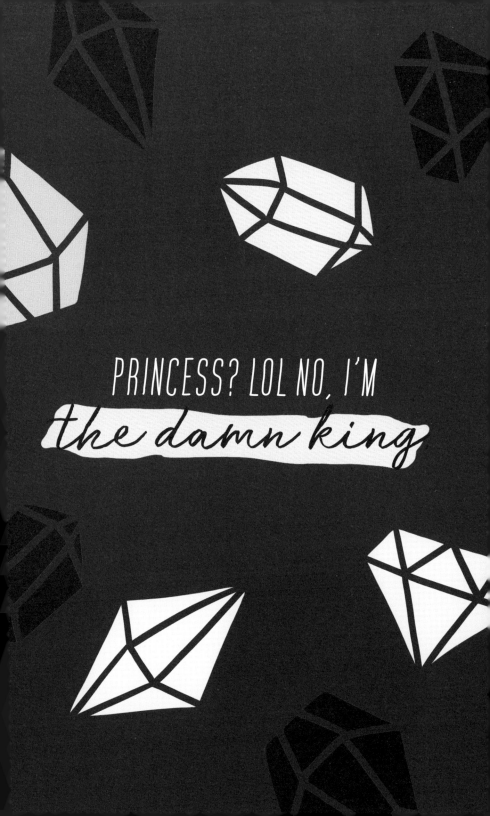

Come up with an internal line you can say to yourself when others get on your last fucking nerve. Tilt your head to the side, smile, and think it real loud.

What is one thing that you can do that others can't?
Celebrate how much of a one-of-a-kind
total badass you are.

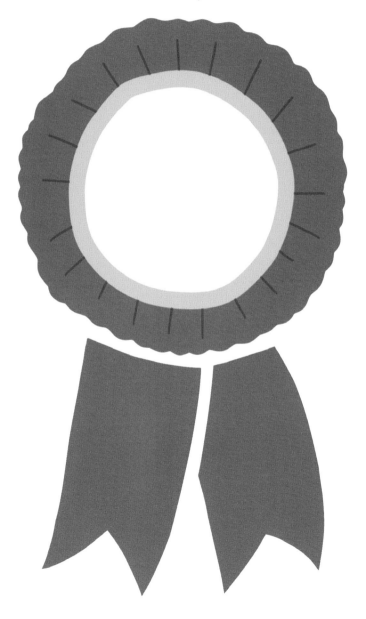

Write about a situation where you held your head high and totally slayed.

What does self-love mean to you?
How can you show yourself some love today?

Repeat this phrase three times:

THAT'S NOT MY FUCKING AGENDA TODAY.

Now describe how you will use it this week.

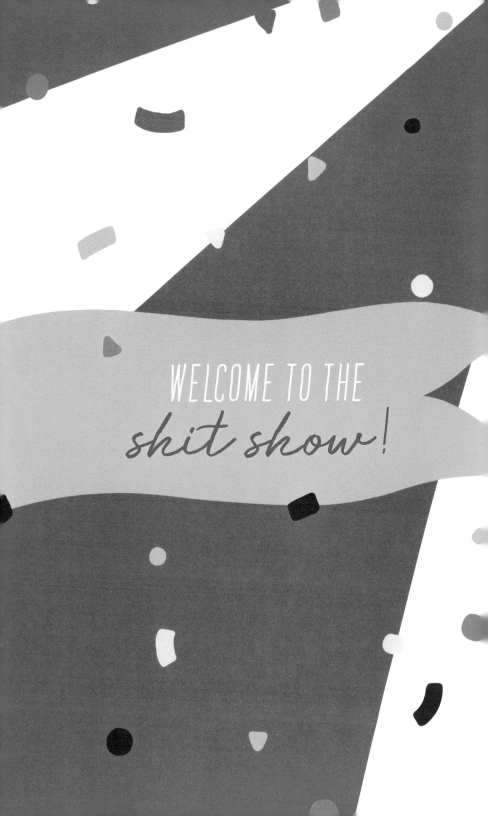

WELCOME TO THE
shit show!

What are some things that bother you that you wish didn't? Rate each one on a scale of one (no problem) to ten (fucking stop it):

- ☐ Sunday paper tossed somewhere along the road.
- ☐ Toothpaste tube squeezed every which way.
- ☐ Being in a group chat where someone says "your" instead of "you're."
- ☐ Waiting a whole fucking afternoon for your laptop to reboot.
- ☐ Realizing you shouldn't have trimmed your hair with all that wine last night.
- ☐ Getting stuck behind a group of slow walkers.
- ☐ Getting all the fucking way to work, then realizing you forgot your laptop at home.
- ☐ Getting interrupted as you're making a really good fucking point.
- ☐ Drivers who toss their trash out of their car windows.
- ☐ Taping the box closed with your Amazon return, then realizing you left out the printed barcode label.
- ☐ Getting showered, dressed, and hair just perfect, then your evening's plans are canceled.
- ☐ Online stores that charge for shipping.
- ☐ "Well, actually..."
- ☐ Couples who sit next to each other in a restaurant booth.
- ☐ A messy, cluttered bedroom/bathroom/kitchen.

Now add up the numbers. The lower your score, the more you are in balance with your "I don't give a shit" inner being.

What does courage mean to you?

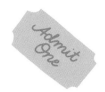

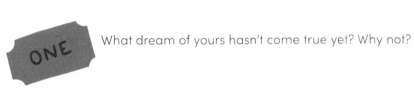
What dream of yours hasn't come true yet? Why not?

Pick one—only one—word that best describes you.

_____

Identify five successes in your life.

KEEP

1 _____

_____

_____

2 _____

_____

_____

3 _____

_____

_____

4 _____

_____

_____

5 _____

_____

_____

WHAT YOU SEE IS *what you fucking get.*

List five people who you feel are good influences in your life. How do they help you be a badass, wonderful, all-around fan-fucking-tastic person?

1 _____

_____

2 _____

_____

3 _____

_____

4 _____

_____

5 _____

_____

What badass quote would you want to be remembered by?

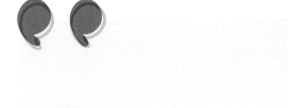

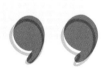

Write down your new secret power word when you are stuck in a situation and need to call up the superbitch in you.

 _____

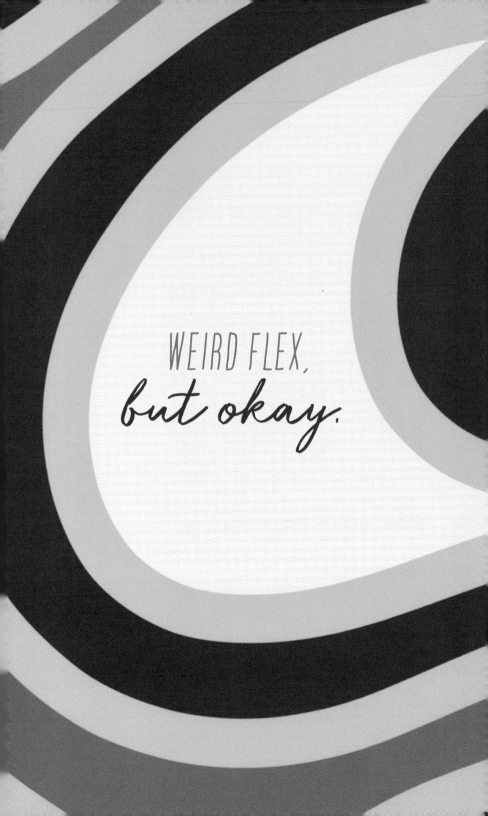

What is one weirdly specific thing you love about yourself?
Like the "I have a freckle in the shape of the state of Michigan"
kind of specific.

Let's say your boss wants you to work on a project you know is outside your pay grade. How do you respond?

_____

_____

_____

_____

_____

_____

_____

_____

What's your "I'm a fucking badass" outfit look like?
This could be anything from tight dresses and stilettos
to baggy shirts and sweatpants.

_____

_____

_____

_____

_____

OH FUCK,
the power
went out.

Fill in the blanks with your favorite sweary words of empowerment and make that shit shine!

I absolutely _____ love myself

because I am so _____ sassy and

badass. My best _____ quality is that

I am _____ strong with a heaping side

of _____ attitude.

Now fill in the blanks with your amazing qualities:

I am so fucking _____ and

_____ that it shines across the

goddamn city. My _____ are fabulous,

my _____ is fan-fucking-tastic, I have

bitchin' _____ and when you see me,

you can't help but say "She's one badass _____

_____."

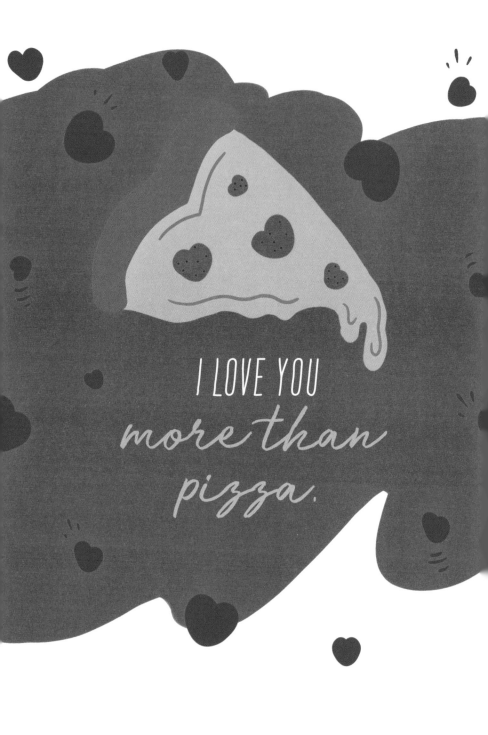

I LOVE YOU
more than
pizza.

Now, write yourself a sappy love letter with all the fixings.
Make it good!

Dear me,

What is the one thing getting in the way of your next goal?
What are you going to do about it?

Circle one of the below statements that now applies to you:

I'm going to be a badass
from this day forward.

I'M GOING TO BE A BADASS
FROM THIS DAY FORWARD.

I'm going to be a badass
from this day forward.

QUIET
that asshole
IN YOUR HEAD

STFU, I'M FOCUSING ON MY MENTAL HEALTH.

True self-care is about paying attention to your mental well-being. Anxiety, stress, depression, all the other emotions and hardships piling up, it can all be a hell of a lot to handle. Self-care helps you take a break from the chaos and focus on your own health. It's about training yourself to not let the bad shit bring you down and celebrating the good in life. It's rewarding yourself for being kind to the number one person around: YOU.

So, take the time to reflect on how your brain is holding up, how your heart is taking it all in. Take a minute and sit with yourself and get to know the good and the bad. Self-care isn't about the external, it isn't something you can throw a filter on and post to your Instagram story. It's about cherishing your well-being, from the inside out. So, get ready, 'cause we're about to shut the negative down and get touchy-feely up in this bitch.

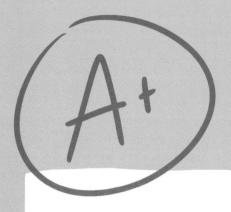

Write down the most recent negative comment you said to yourself.

_____

_____

_____

_____

_____

Now throw it the fuck away because you're never going to say it again.

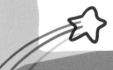

Which are the various types of self-care?

A. Psychological
B. Spiritual
C. Emotional
D. Physical
E. Professional
F. A and B but not C
G. B and C but not A
H. All except F and G
I. A through E but not F
J. These multiple choices are giving me damn flashbacks

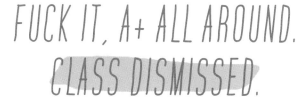

FUCK IT, A+ ALL AROUND.
CLASS DISMISSED.

What one thing are you never ever ever fucking ever going to do again?

_____

_____

_____

_____

_____

_____

_____

_____

_____

_____

_____

_____

_____

How does stress and anxiety manifest in your life?
What's your go-to anxiety-relieving activity?

_____

_____

_____

_____

_____

_____

_____

_____

_____

_____

_____

_____

_____

Let's play the opposite game: You know those days when you just want to hide away from people and life in general? Fuck that. Go for the opposite of what you are feeling. Need to isolate? Put on your shoes and that cute new top and head to the mall, a crowded store, or a busy park. Just soak in your time around people. Describe what that felt like.

Think of one person in your life—whether a spouse, partner, coworker, or family member—who embodies self-empowerment. What traits does this person have, and how can you adopt one of those traits for yourself?

Identify five emotions you experienced today.

1 _____

2 _____

3 _____

4 _____

5 _____

Of those five emotions, which one was the hardest to deal with? Why?

Describe the steps you perform for a favorite ritual, whether it's preparing tea, setting up movie night, or getting ready to go out for the evening. How does that routine make you feel?

WINNER WINNER
chicken dinner

Check off a few ways you will reward yourself for just making it through the goddamn month:

Buy that pricey sweater you wanted.
Stop at the ice cream aisle and power move one right into the damn cart.
Go through your pile of unread books and get reading.
Upgrade your iPhone.
Get some flowers from the market and fill your living room.
Dig out a comfy old shirt and wear it out in public.
Look through your Amazon wish list and slide an item into your cart.
Write up a positive review for yourself that reflects how you traveled through the month.
Invite a friend over and just stalk Insta profiles all night.
Get a candle going, fill the tub, and hop in with a nothing-having-to-do-with-reality magazine.
Download a new game app on your phone. Start playing!
Pile up some clothes you haven't worn in a year and donate them. Start fresh!
Clean out the kitchen cupboards. Hey, it works for some people.

What do you think are some differences between psychological and emotional self-care?

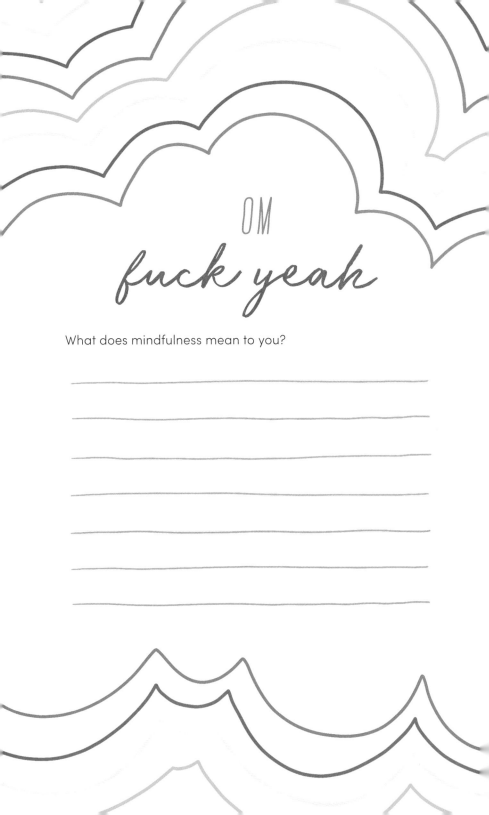

OM
fuck yeah

What does mindfulness mean to you?

_____

_____

_____

_____

_____

_____

_____

Describe a situation recently where you practiced mindfulness and didn't even realize you were doing it!

Have you done something positive and forgot to congratulate yourself? Why the fuck did you do that? Now's your chance to write up a note to your awesome self.

What have you done or felt that surprised you this past month?

Remember the last time you were so goddamn happy?
Describe the situation and your surroundings at the time.

IT'S
my party
AND I'LL CRY IF I
fucking want to

Do you have a happy place? What does it look like?

_____

_____

_____

_____

_____

_____

_____

_____

_____

_____

_____

_____

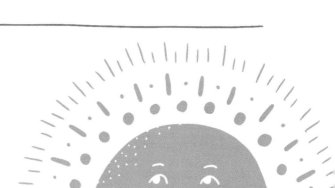

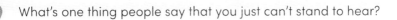

What's one thing people say that you just can't stand to hear?

One in five adults will experience mental illness this year **(Nami.org)**. How can you help out a friend who is struggling?

Describe one shitty thing that happened to you this month.

Now rewrite it so that it has a positive lesson.

Close your eyes and sit quietly for five minutes.
What were some thoughts that raced around in your head?

DIVE INTO THE EMOTION OCEAN

How emotionally intelligent are you?

I can find the right word to describe how I'm feeling.
A. Yes
B. Sometimes, occasionally, frequently, well maybe periodically.
C. No

I can tell exactly what my friend is feeling.
A. Yes
B. Only if she's pissed. You really need to see it.
C. No

I can tell the difference between anger and frustration.
A. Yes
B. Goddamn it I just can't right now.
C. No

I manipulate another's feelings.
A. No way.
B. I'm feeling bad about this one. Did you make me feel bad on purpose?
C. Aw, but it's so easy.

I am free to share how I feel with others.
A. Hell, I may even show them this journal.
B. When things are going great, sure.
C. No one wants to know how I feel.

Answers
If you picked mostly A's, you are fucking emotion smart.
If you picked mostly B's, you have a bit of work to do on that emotional IQ.
If you picked mostly C's, oh, honey, bless your heart. Go back to page 1 of this journal.

Mental health awareness is crucial, not just for you but for your loved ones as well. Check off any signs you've noticed in yourself or a loved one.

- Avoiding friends or social situations
- Constant worry or fear
- Extreme and persistent feelings of sadness
- Change in school performance
- Drastic change in sleeping or eating habits
- Substance abuse
- Unable to perform daily tasks
- Loss of interest in hobbies and passions
- Thoughts of self-harm or suicide

For more information, warning signs, and how to get help, visit **Nami.org**.

Now write this on a sticky note and paste it on your mirror:

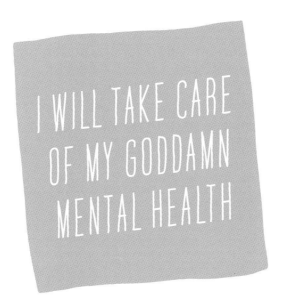

BITCH,
just do what feels good!

WHAT'S A GOOD HABIT? SOMETHING THAT MAKES YOU ACTUALLY FEEL BETTER!

We all want to be badass humans with skins of steel who only eat organic vegetables handpicked from the remote plains and always make their damn beds in the morning. Because, we're told those good habits are supposed to make us better people. But guess what, sometimes, it's okay to break your routine, let the shit in, and embrace the "bad" in your life. In fact, sometimes it can be the best thing for you.

Every once in a while screaming in your car or crying on your living room couch feels really fucking good. A glass of wine at the end of the day can feel good, going out with your friends until 3:00 a.m. can feel good. Falling asleep at 8:00 p.m. can be just what you need and eating an entire bag of tortilla chips can be the healthiest thing you do (at least for your soul). At the end of the day, guess what? None of these habits, done sparingly, are hurting you long term. Give yourself the space to feel good without that voice in your head nagging at you that you're not doing everything "right." Instead, embrace the curves life throws you, listen to your heart and your body, and do what actually feels good!

This is an opportunity to stop the holier-than-thou self-care culture and actually lean in to your potential. Find what helps you cope with and excel at life. Discover how to serve others. And most importantly, discover how to serve yourself.

So, in conclusion, stop with the bad habit, regimented-as-hell bullshit, and just DO WHAT FEELS FUCKING GOOD.

What are five things that always make you feel good as hell?

1 --

----

2 --

----

3 --

----

4 --

----

5 --

What three things are you really really good at?

1 --

----

2 --

----

3 --

STOP BEING A JERKY MCJERKFACE

How much of a bully is your inner critic?
Circle which of these statements reflects your inner critic:

There's a party Friday night:
A. They probably won't invite me.
B. I'm not sure I'll look as good as everyone else there.
C. There sure is and it's at MY house, goddamn it.

What a fucky, gloomy day:
A. My friends won't want to hear my lame problems.
B. I'm sure it's my fault the weather sucks.
C. Gloomy? This is what I call pre-Halloween! Yes!

I need three more credits this semester:
A. I'm not smart enough to take that higher-level class.
B. Everyone will be smarter than me in the class.
C. Registered. Done.

Answers
If you chose A's, your inner critic is a goddamn bully. Stop it.
If you chose B's, you're trying. Let's work on trying harder.
If you chose C's, your inner critic may be lurking but YOU are the boss!

⚡ GUILTY AS CHARGED ⚡

Make a list of your top ten guilty pleasures.

1 _____

2 _____

3 _____

4 _____

5 _____

6 _____

7 _____

8 _____

9 _____

10 _____

Now cross off the word "guilty" and circle the word "pleasures."

DROP THE BUCKET LIST.
IT'S TIME FOR A FUCK-IT LIST!

Which of these activities will you say fuck it and try this week, even if you don't have the time? Yes, you do have to pick at least one:

- Bring a cup of coffee or tea back to bed and read that book that's been sitting on your bedside table. Stay there until the coffee is done.
- Stay in your pajamas all damn day.
- Listen to your favorite album with the volume all the way up.
- Cry, just because you want to.
- Watch YouTube videos of cute animals for at least an hour.
- Order the venti latte because you deserve it.
- Get on the phone with a friend and talk for a solid hour.
- Sleep in until noon.
- Have ice cream for dinner. Just ice cream.
- No texting. For at least an hour.
- Instagram at least five outdoor photos.
- Rent something new on Redbox even though you have Netflix.
- Say that argument you've been bottling up for so long, just to get it all out.
- Take a nap in the middle of the afternoon.
- All of these. Do all of these.

Write down a quick feel-good phrase you can use this week for something you are not looking forward to.

Find ten minutes today to do absolutely nothing. Lie in the grass with your arms and legs spread out like a starfish. C'mon, just ten fucking minutes. How did that feel? Could you do it?

_____

_____

_____

_____

_____

_____

_____

_____

_____

_____

_____

_____

_____

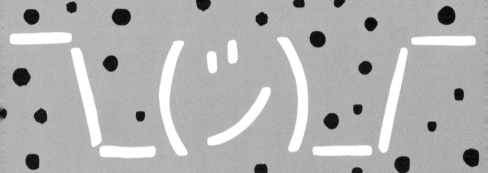

feeling

IDGAF-ISH TODAY

What did you do this week that you felt you probably shouldn't have?

Now cut that shit out. Who needs fucking negativity anyway.

Describe a recent time when you just wanted to sit on the couch and cry.

Now tell yourself you fucking needed it, so who the fuck cares.

Doing things for others feels just as good as doing things for ourselves. If you had a free day next week, what community service project would you want to try?

What's your favorite dessert?

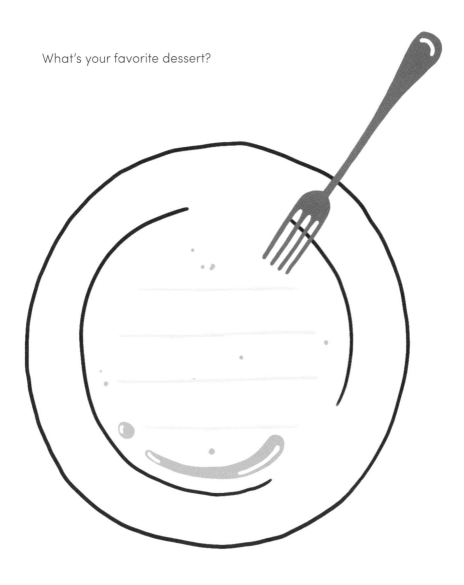

Yum. Now go ahead and have it before dinner today.
Why the fuck not?

What's your normal bedtime?

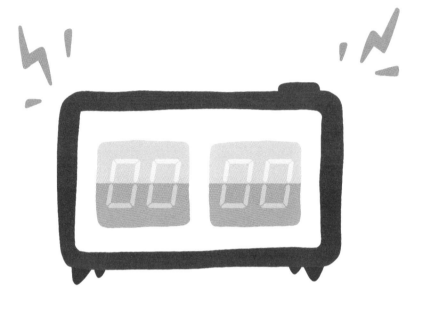

Are you fucking serious? Go to bed at nine tonight just for the hell of it. How did that feel?

Do you remember your nighttime cuddly toy?
What are you carrying around as an adult that gives
you that same sense of security?

_____

_____

_____

_____

_____

_____

_____

_____

_____

_____

_____

_____

_____

_____

What did you do this month that set you off into fits of giggles? Make that your weekly medicine.

_____

_____

_____

_____

_____

_____

_____

_____

_____

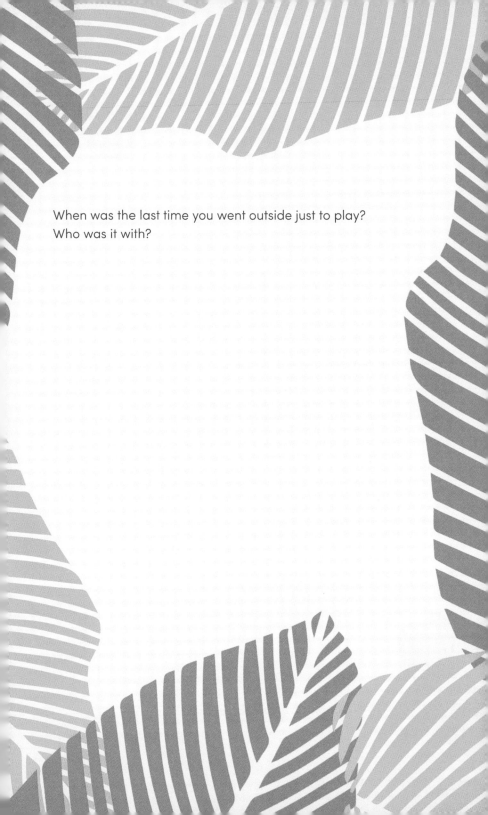

When was the last time you went outside just to play?
Who was it with?

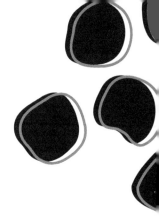

Sometimes you just need to let it out.
What five curse words or phrases do you use?

1 _____

_____

2 _____

_____

3 _____

_____

4 _____

_____

5 _____

_____

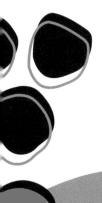

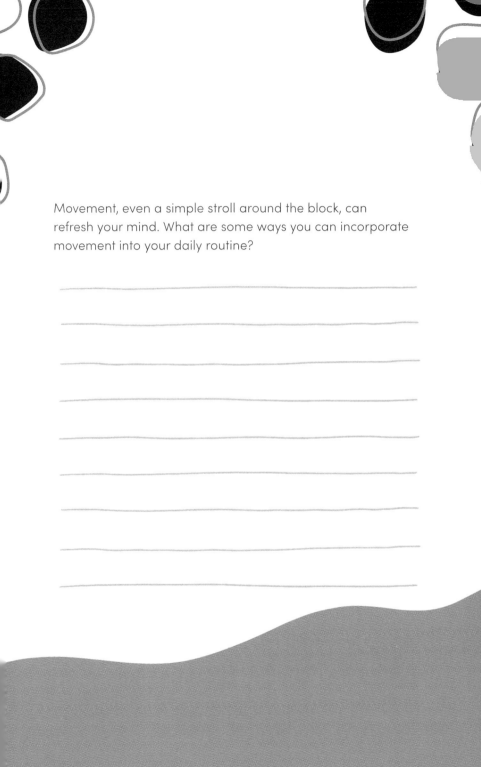

Movement, even a simple stroll around the block, can refresh your mind. What are some ways you can incorporate movement into your daily routine?

_____

_____

_____

_____

_____

_____

_____

_____

WE DO THE
monster mask

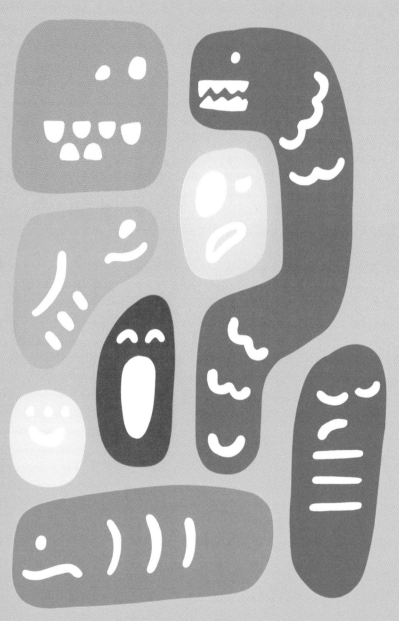

Some days can be overwhelming. If you feel that goddamn panic monster rising up, stop what you are doing and check off the following to keep that monster at bay:

- One thing colorful you can see

- One sound that is pleasant

- A lovely smell outside

- Taste something (what do you mean you forgot to bring that chocolate?)

- Touch two different textures and describe them

Who are the people in your life you can go to for advice?

_____

_____

_____

_____

_____

_____

_____

_____

GROW THE
complimen-tree

Write down at least ten self-compliments.
Make them fucking good!

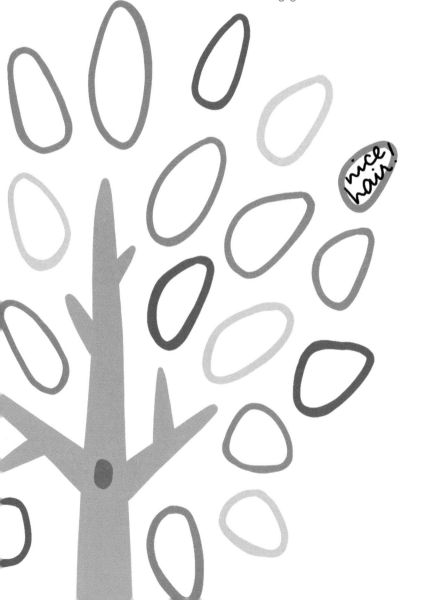

nice hair!

What is your definition of "fun"?

What brings you joy? Not just fun but pure fucking joy.

How long do you stay at a party if you are not having fun?
What is your exit strategy?

_____

_____

_____

Today you are feeling both
powerful and self-aware.
Come up with a T-shirt
slogan to reflect that.

(   )   -

Which friend would be a good self-care buddy for those
days that you just can't get through? Write down the name
and number. Keep this handy and call that person this month!

How do you handle things when bad shit happens?

_____

_____

_____

_____

_____

_____

_____

For some stupid-ass reason, your boss rejected your project.
Do you:
A. Stalk the fucker.
B. Who needs that shit? There's a better idea on the way.

You've been unfriended. Do you:
A. Stalk the fucker.
B. Post the happiest photos of you having the best time.

A friend has been sharing untrue info about you. Do you:
A. Stalk the fucker.
B. Send her flowers for upping your popularity

Your partner is having feelings for your best friend. Do you:
A. Stalk the fucker (both of them).
B. They may be happy together, who knows. Who cares?

Answers
If you chose even one A, we need to work on a few things.
If you chose all B's, sell some of that power in a jar, you fucking star!

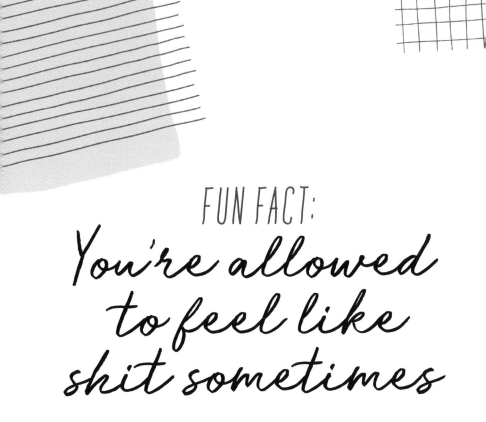

FUN FACT:
You're allowed to feel like shit sometimes

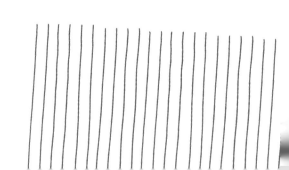

x x x x

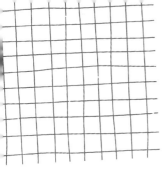

BECAUSE EMOTIONAL INTELLIGENCE IS WOKE AF

Sometimes, no matter what we do, we're just going to feel like shit. And guess what, that's okay! We all get in those moods, we all stumble into those pitfalls, and we all have to wade through life's tsunamis. What you have to remember is: it always gets fucking better. And in the meantime, you can learn how to grow and move forward like the badass you are.

When you've hit a rough patch, give yourself the space to be sad and try to discover the patterns in your mood. Sometimes feeling bad is fucking necessary. And sometimes it even feels really damn good. Watch a movie that makes you cry. Yell out all the things that have been bottling inside. Rage at the universe and tell them they're not playing fucking fair. Just remember, we all go through the storms, and in the end, they make us stronger and more amazing than we ever would've known.

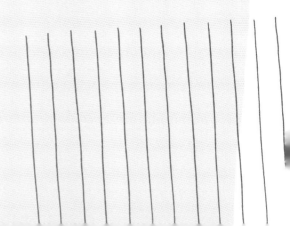

Describe what it feels like when nothing seems to be going your way.

Describe a situation this month when you felt like you couldn't handle things.

Now write down what happened afterward. What did you do?

What is one habit you have that just irritates the hell out of you?

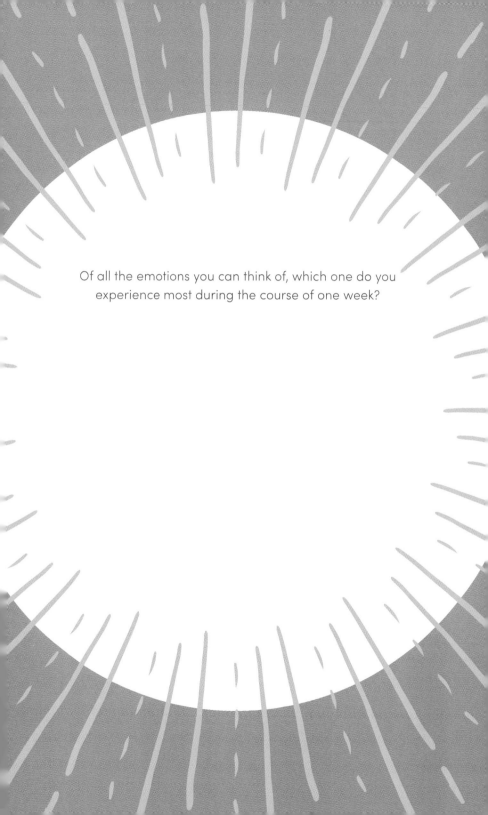

Of all the emotions you can think of, which one do you experience most during the course of one week?

Did you ever want to be a character from a book you've read? Who and why?

What are three go-to movies you can watch when your week
just sucks and you need to get out of your problems for a bit?

1 _____

2 _____

3 _____

HOLLYWOOD
walk of shame

Check off any of the movie titles that reflect how you feel when your week is shitty as fuck:

- [ ] Sleepless in Seattle
- [ ] Throw Momma from the Train
- [ ] Miss Congeniality
- [ ] Desperado
- [ ] Walking Tall
- [ ] The Hangover
- [ ] Gone in 60 Seconds
- [ ] Harry Potter and the Prisoner of Azkaban
- [ ] Psycho
- [ ] Little Miss Sunshine
- [ ] Home Alone
- [ ] Dumb and Dumber
- [ ] Gone with the Wind
- [ ] Rebel without a Cause
- [ ] A Star is Born
- [ ] Stranger than Fiction
- [ ] Freaky Friday
- [ ] Mamma Mia! Here We Go Again!
- [ ] Avengers: Endgame

Crappy day? What's a good book title that best describes your situation?

_____

_____

_____

I DON'T KNOW HER...

Draw a picture of your morning face.

morning face

Now draw a picture of your morning face not giving
a fuck about yesterday's problems.

NO FUCKS
morning face

How many times this month have you spoken negatively about yourself? What did you say?

_____

_____

_____

_____

_____

_____

_____

Now take those negative phrases and rewrite them here in a positive way.

_____

_____

_____

_____

_____

_____

_____

C'EST LA

fucking vie

If your best friend is having a shitty day and needs your support, how do you comfort them?

_____

_____

_____

_____

_____

_____

_____

_____

_____

_____

_____

_____

_____

Identify a surefire way that would comfort YOU the next time your day goes to hell.

_____

_____

_____

_____

_____

_____

_____

_____

_____

_____

_____

_____

Emotional intelligence includes being aware of and identifying your emotions, harnessing and using them effectively, and managing control over them.

Match the term with the definition:
A. awareness
B. harness
C. management

☐ **1.** I can easily tell when my friend is depressed.
☐ **2.** Sure I'm pissed, but I've got on a hell of a smile.
☐ **3.** This heart pounding is probably anxiety.
☐ **4.** Get out of my damn lane! Nice signal ya got there!
☐ **5.** This won't be fun, but dammit I'm going to slow-breathe all the way through it.

Answers: 1. A; 2. C; 3. A; 4. B; 5. C

Your score:
Five correct: You are an Einstein of emotional IQ.
Four correct: You're right up there with Einstein's cat.
Three or less correct: Okay, so maybe you don't have emotional intelligence; we're working on it.

CHUMP CHANGE

Stop being a pushover. Write out five ways you can assert yourself and start earning back that chump change.

1 _____

_____

2 _____

_____

3 _____

_____

4 _____

_____

5 _____

_____

What would you do if someone significant makes a decision for you, but you don't really think it's what's best?

Do you consider yourself brave?
What do you think it means to be brave?

What's the funniest thing that happened to you this week?

How do you handle anger?

What's the difference between anger and frustration?

Not everyone takes the same sized steps to reach goals.
What small steps can you celebrate today?

What one struggle or challenge can you just let go of? Great.
Now, let it go. And you're welcome for that song in your ear now.

Describe one emotion that you wish you'd never have to feel again. Why? What emotion is its opposite? What do they both have in common?

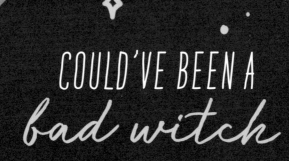

COULD'VE BEEN A
bad witch

We all love a popular self-care routine. But what if you want to just go fucking nonstandard and do something a bit more magical? See how many of these you can do over the next month. Go on. Get out of your fucking comfort zone.

Light a candle, then sit and stare at it for ten minutes.

Burn some incense and float it around the room, *Practical Magic* style.

Stand tall, arms outstretched, and pretend you are a tree with your feet as roots.

Go to a park and spend twenty minutes on the swing.

Bring your dinner outside and eat it on a blanket in the grass.

Rearrange a room in your home.

Spend an hour just watching funny pet videos.

Make it through an entire yoga video.

Plant an herb, then check on it every day. Don't forget to play in the dirt.

Get a few essential oils and try to come up with a new aroma blend.

Head to the craft store and get a bead kit. Make gifts!

Subscribe to free sign language videos. Then use that new skill!

Start a local meetup group with a hobby you've wanted to try.

Borrow a free library audiobook on guided meditation and take a mental trip.

Go through a boring chore (such as washing dishes) with mindfulness. What's the water temperature? How does the soap feel? How heavy are the plates? Is your posture strong? Are you washing in a pattern or haphazard? Slow it down. Feel it.

FEELING SOME TYPE OF WAY

So, how do you feel about showcasing your emotions?

You just finished an exhausting crying spell. Do you:
A. fall immediately asleep and hope to wake up refreshed.
B. head to the kitchen for a treat.
C. wash your face and get your ass outside.

You are driving to work and crying over an emotional song.
A car pulls up beside you at the light. You:
A. hide your face from the driver.
B. point to the radio and smile.
C. slide down your window and ask for tissue.

At a restaurant, you overhear a customer bullying a server. You:
A. shake your head and say "Bless her heart."
B. leave an extra large tip for her suffering.
C. head over to the table and tell the bastard "That was my
   sister on her first day working after a terrible illness.
   I hope you were supportive."

Answers
If you picked A's, you don't have time for emotions.
If you picked B's, you accept your emotions but prefer to hide them.
If you picked C's, you fucking OWN it.

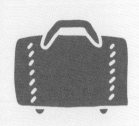
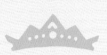

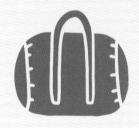

GET UP AND HANDLE
your fucking business

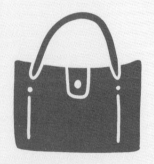
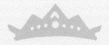

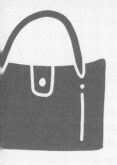
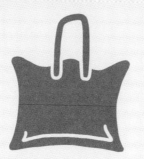

WEAR YOUR EMPOWERMENT LIKE A DAMN CROWN

Self-care is not an excuse to ignore the demands of your life. You're not going to sit in a bubble bath and lounge in athleisure instead of going to work and getting shit done. Even if we sometimes want to ignore our piling to-do list, we can't always, and self-care isn't an excuse to give up. Repeat after me: it's not about letting things slide; it's about advocating for what you truly want.

It's time to stand up and demand the things that will bring you joy. You deserve that raise? Then you go make it happen. You feel underappreciated? Then stand up and say something. If you're adrift in the world, it's because you haven't discovered your purpose. Because purpose is the ultimate tenet of true self-care. It's about making the world a better place for tomorrow, both for yourself and for everyone around you. So, get ready to step out of your comfort zone, charge forward, and seize the fucking day.

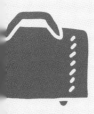

List all the things that went right today.

_____

_____

_____

_____

_____

_____

_____

_____

_____

_____

_____

_____

_____

_____

_____

If your boss said you were not going to get a raise this year, write down your plan of action to counteract his dumbass decision.

_____

_____

_____

_____

_____

_____

_____

_____

_____

_____

_____

_____

_____

_____

Go out this week and hold the door open to three random strangers. What were their reactions?

1 _____

_____

2 _____

_____

3 _____

_____

Visit the library and volunteer to read aloud a children's book to unsuspecting kids. Were they grateful? How did that go? You did check with the parents first, right?

_____

_____

_____

_____

_____

_____

You have a shitty meeting coming up and need help getting out the door. The night before, set out sticky notes starting from your bedroom to the coffeepot to the shower to the fridge, then one on the door. What energizing messages will you write on those notes?

What appointments have you been putting off? Dental?
Vision? Lab work? Make those calls this week and place
a check next to it when you're done.

- [ ] _____
- [ ] _____
- [ ] _____
- [ ] _____
- [ ] _____
- [ ] _____
- [ ] _____
- [ ] _____
- [ ] _____
- [ ] _____
- [ ] _____
- [ ] _____
- [ ] _____
- [ ] _____
- [ ] _____

Open up your calendar. Pick a day. Now add in something fun for you to do that is not work or chore related. Come back to this day and fill in the star here if you actually went out and had fun!

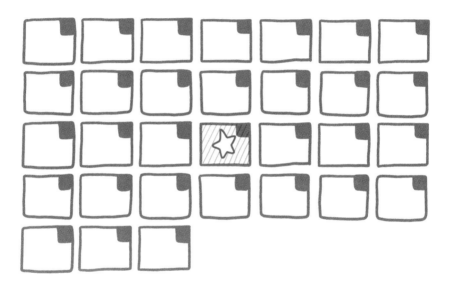

LIKE A

DAMN BOSS

What activity coming up are you dreading? Why?
(If it's an office retreat, we totally understand.)

_____

_____

_____

_____

_____

_____

_____

You have two equally fun Friday-night invitations.
What process do you use to select which one you will choose?

_____

_____

_____

_____

_____

_____

_____

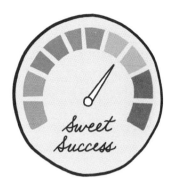

SUCCESS-O-METER

You have a gratitude list, right? (Of course you do.)
How about a success list? Go on—make a list of your top
ten successes of all time to push that meter to the max:

1 _____

2 _____

3 _____

4 _____

5 _____

6 _____

7 _____

8 _____

9 _____

10 _____

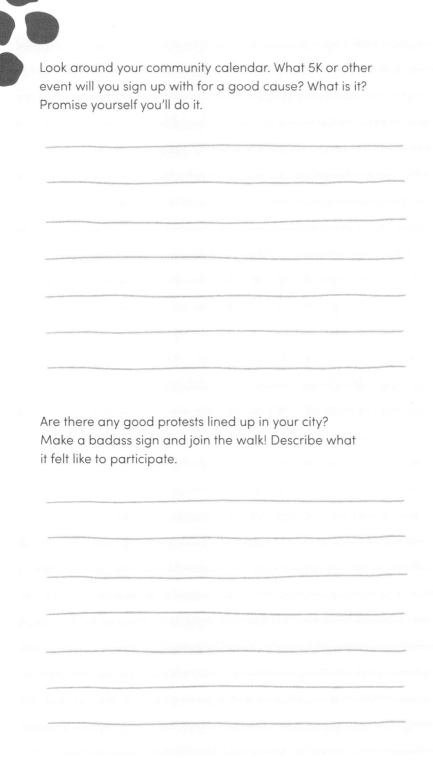

Look around your community calendar. What 5K or other event will you sign up with for a good cause? What is it? Promise yourself you'll do it.

_____

_____

_____

_____

_____

_____

Are there any good protests lined up in your city? Make a badass sign and join the walk! Describe what it felt like to participate.

_____

_____

_____

_____

_____

_____

Write a draft letter here to a senator about how he royally fucked up. Are you brave enough to send it?

YOU DID THAT ON PURPOSE!

What does purpose mean to you? Have you discovered
what your purpose is?

_____

_____

_____

_____

_____

_____

_____

_____

_____

_____

What are three goals that serve your purpose?

1 _____

2 _____

3 _____

What about passion? What are you passionate about?

It's time to go to the dreaded DMV. How can you make the long-ass wait more bearable before tearing your goddamn hair out?

How safe is your neighborhood? What can you do to feel more safe? Petition for a streetlight? Corner crossing signs? Write down the plan, then get on it!

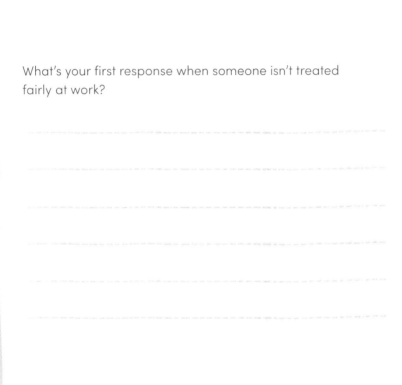

What's your first response when someone isn't treated fairly at work?

You are signed up for a class, bought the textbook,
but a week into the class you hate it. What do you do?

Do you have a to-do list a goddamn mile long? What are the top five items on it?

1 _____

2 _____

3 _____

4 _____

5 _____

Now circle just one you'll get done today.

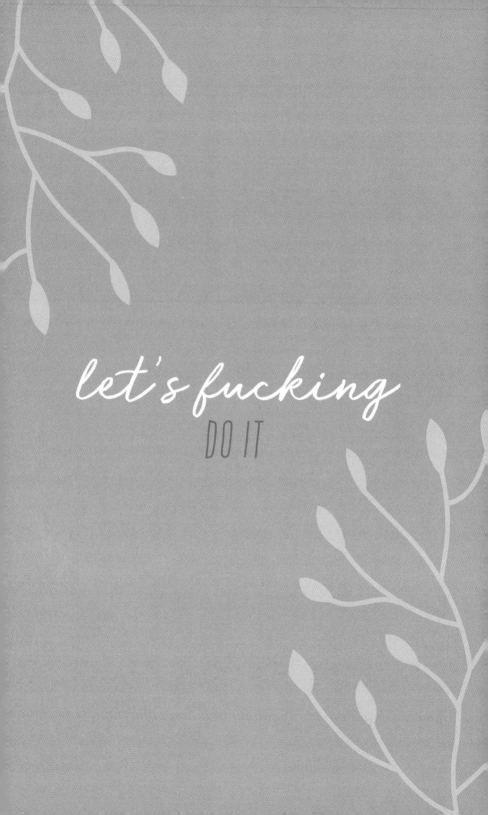

Three of your friends want you to go to the movies with them. How do you convince them to see the movie YOU want to see?

_____

_____

_____

_____

_____

_____

_____

_____

It's another shitty day at work. Prepare an argument to your boss for why you need to take the afternoon off for a mindful walk.

_____

_____

_____

_____

_____

_____

_____

_____

_____

_____

_____

_____

_____

_____

What is one artistic or soothing endeavor you can commit to today that'll make the world a better place?

How did you feel creating?

You have prescriptions to pick up, groceries to get, a pet to pick up from the vet, and a thousand other things. Write out a strategy to get it all done with enough time for that glass of wine and a new book that you managed to somehow get while you were out doing every other goddamn thing. Yay you!

chill pill

ALL RIGHT,
*calm the
fuck down!*

**All that power and badassery is exhausting.
Don't forget to restore and refresh. Check these
off when you've tried each one.**

- Sat outside in the morning with a cup of coffee or tea. Oh, and actually enjoyed the entire cup, not just a hurried sip and dash. You know who you are.

- Sat through an entire movie...with popcorn. Um, who watches a movie without popcorn?

- Browsed a bookstore...just because. Bonus points for actually buying a book. And a truckload of chocolate is headed your way if you sat down to read the damn thing.

- Played music while brushing your dog or cat. Or a neighbor's cat. Yeah, you should probably get permission first.

What will motivate you to get off the couch when you really just want to lie there all damn night, soaking in your bad day?

_____

_____

_____

_____

_____

A family member calls and starts whining on and on and fucking on, but you just added a movie to the queue and the cookies are fresh from the oven. What will you say when you answer the phone?

_____

_____

_____

_____

_____

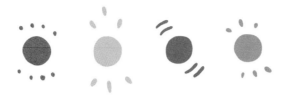

PARENTAL CONTROLS

Your mom comes to visit for the weekend. When you get home from work on Friday, she has cheerfully rearranged all the living room and bedroom furniture and put shell and flamingo decorations in your bathroom.
Choose your best response:

A. Pack up and move. Now.

B. Paste on a smile and tell her it's lovely.

C. Stand in the middle of each room and bawl your fucking head off.

D. Give her ten bucks to go get a coffee, then put everything back in its place.

E. Why was your mom alone in your house? You know what she's capable of.

Answer: There's no right answer. You shouldn't have given her the key to get in.

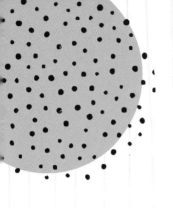

STOP
giving a fuck!

FINALLY DITCH THE ANXIETY OF SAYING NO

You know what, people can be really fucking draining. We love them, we love to be around them, but sometimes it's time to step back and refocus on your own well-being. After a long week, when that third invitation for drinks with Chatty Kathy comes your way, just say no. When your BFF tries to throw you into the drama wringer with her latest gossip binge, follow up with a nope, not today. And when your ex comes crawling back asking for a stress-filled, emotional landmine riddled talk sesh, you can politely tell them to fuck off. Because the number one person you need to look out for is YOU, and it's totally okay to stop the bullshit and walk away.

Finally ditch the anxiety of saying no! Boundaries are an important tenet of self-care, so draw them! It's not being a bitch, it's about standing up for your time and being an advocate for your own wellness.

So, stop giving fucks. Stop giving fucks to people who drain you, who ask things of you and do not reciprocate. Set boundaries on your friendships, your obligations, your personal time. Learn when to say yes and when to say no. But even more, learn to be okay saying no.

OH NO!
YOU'RE ALMOST OUT OF FUCKS!

**You've only got five fucks to give but ten problems.
Check off which five you'll use those fuck tickets on.**

- ☐ Your neighbor is blasting heavy metal as you're trying to sleep.

- ☐ You find your first gray hair.

- ☐ You get ghosted by your latest dating app crush.

- ☐ Your roommate ate the leftovers you were saving.

- ☐ You dropped your last contact lens down the sink.

- ☐ The power went out just as you were blow-drying your hair.

- ☐ You ran out of gas halfway to work.

- ☐ Your friend is guilt tripping you to go to a terrible bar you hate.

- ☐ All your phone apps suddenly uninstalled.

- ☐ You accidentally sent that practice sweary email to your professor or boss.

Life is going to happen no matter what you can do about it.

Try radical acceptance (RA). Say: *Yes it's going to happen. Yes I can prepare for it.*

Then add your RA phrase: *But I don't have to plaster a goddamn smile on my face about it.*

Now come up with your own RA phrase for when the shit hits the fan.

ENTER THE
douche canoe

Fill the canoe with all the douchebag things people have asked of you and finally flip that fucker over.

_____

_____

_____

_____

_____

_____

Do you have an inner critic? What was the most recent thing that dumbass said to you?

_____

_____

_____

_____

_____

_____

What are some kick-ass phrases you can say to that bully of an inner critic?

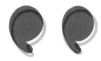

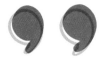

Now let's give it a name. Make it a horrible, ugly-ass nasty but funny name. Write it down. Say it. Say it with scorn!

_____

_____

_____

_____

_____

_____

_____

What are five boring chores or errands this week
that you can ignore and not give a shit about?

1 ———————————————————————————

2 ———————————————————————————

3 ———————————————————————————

4 ———————————————————————————

5 ———————————————————————————

DEFEND THE FUCKING FORTRESS

It's time to draw those boundaries. Draw the impenetrable walls that'll keep you away from all the bullshit. What are you using to defend your castle of stay the fuck away?

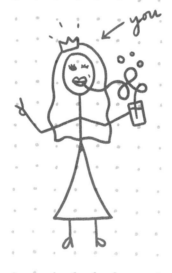

In what five situations this past month did you say yes
when you should have said no?

1 _____

_____

2 _____

_____

3 _____

_____

4 _____

_____

5 _____

_____

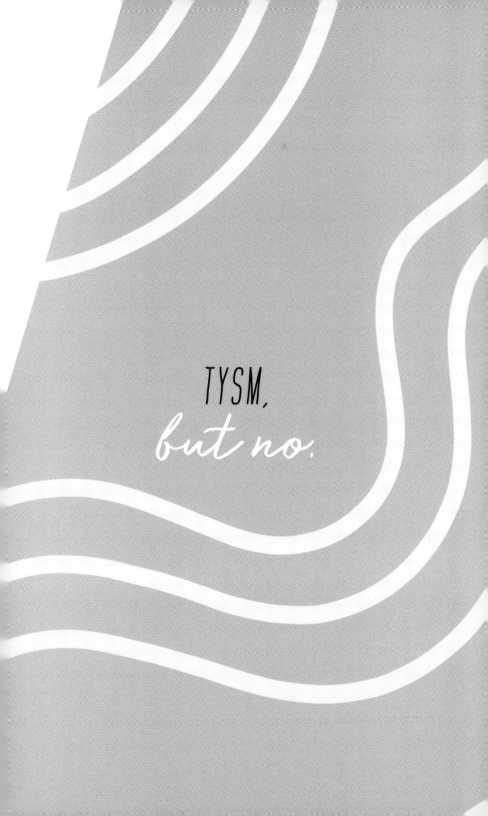

TYSM,
but no.

What would you do if someone keeps interrupting you during a conversation?

Your friends are planning a party and somehow you've gotten stuck doing all the grunt work. How do you confront the situation?

What's a past mistake you've made that you haven't been able to let go of? Can you do it now?

Your most recent ex texted you saying they want to talk, but you know the conversation is going to be emotionally draining. How do you handle it?

CUE
the dramatics

Circle the correct answer. What would you say if someone told you to "Quit making a scene"?

A. Oops, my bad.

B. Sorry I embarrassed you.

C. I'll whisper now.

D. You're right. I was wrong.

E. Sorry, let's focus on you now.

F. I'll just slink away to another room.

G. Scene? I'll show you a goddamn scene with a full fucking plot!

The answer is you goddamn better know the correct answer by now.

fuck

GIVE-A-FUCK JAR

Write down the word *fuck* on
five note cards, then put them
in a jar. That's all you get for
the month. After you used
them, tell everyone your "give
a fuck" jar is empty and they'll
have to wait until next month.

Your night is ready. Tea, snacks, new book, fresh-from-the-dryer pj's, cool evening. But two friends want to come over for a bitch session. How are those boundaries looking?

_____

_____

_____

_____

_____

_____

Have you ever been in a situation where you just wanted to yell "I don't give a fuck!" and walk away? What was the situation and how could you have taken more control of it?

_____

_____

_____

_____

_____

_____

ABSO-FUCKING-LUTELY
not.

What three things did you recently say yes to that you wish you hadn't?

1 _____

_____

2 _____

_____

3 _____

_____

Develop an award-winning phrase to use when you just want to be alone for a while.

Now write up one you know your friend could really use. Wrap it up and gift it!

What is one thing you wish people would stop pestering you about?

HOW "ON" IS YOUR
I don't give a shit
METER?

A. I don't give a shit, but I'll do it anyway.

B. I don't give a shit, and if I wait long enough it will go away.

C. I don't give a shit. Neither should you.

D. I don't give a shit. Let's do something else.

E. I don't fucking give a shit, end of story.

Answers
If you picked A, you need to practice. In the car, at home, at the store.
If you picked B, your meter is passive-aggressive.
If you picked C, your meter wants a friend.
If you picked D, your meter is a pro at changing the subject.
If you picked E, there ya go!

What's one criticism you hear that fucking bothers you?
Write your ideal response to it.

_____

_____

_____

_____

_____

_____

_____

Do some friends drain your energy? Why do you think that is?

_____

_____

_____

_____

_____

_____

_____

Which TV character is most like you? Why?

_____

_____

_____

_____

_____

_____

_____

What's one of your character traits you'd like to no longer have? Can you do something about that?

What's the first thing you will say to yourself as soon as you wake up in the morning?

You are now an expert at standing up for your own self-care. Write down your NOPE response for each of these scenarios. Say it loud. Say it fucking strong!

Can I stay over at your place for a week?

That class is full, but we're sure you'll like this one better.

Can you watch my cat for a couple of weeks?

Do you have time to take me to the airport at 5:00 a.m.?

This is delicious wine. Let's trim each other's hair tonight!

Can I borrow your laptop and take it to a coffee shop?

Let's take a two-month RV trip across the U.S.!

You can no longer have chocolate.

now you're f*cking radiant

TRACK YOUR SELF-CARE AND SHOW OFF HOW YOU GOT TO YOUR FAN-FUCKING-TASTIC SELF!

Self-care is an ongoing journey, so track your progress in your own self-care log. Fill out the week on the left and write in the self-care techniques you use each day, then at the end, rate your fucking radiance on a scale of 1–10.

DATE RANGE		
MO		
TU		
WE		
TH		
FR		
SA		
SU		
RADIANCE SCORE		

DATE RANGE		
MO		
TU		
WE		
TH		
FR		
SA		
SU		
RADIANCE SCORE		

DATE RANGE		
MO		
TU		
WE		
TH		
FR		
SA		
SU		
RADIANCE SCORE		

DATE RANGE		
MO		
TU		
WE		
TH		
FR		
SA		
SU		
RADIANCE SCORE		

DATE RANGE		
MO		
TU		
WE		
TH		
FR		
SA		
SU		
RADIANCE SCORE		

DATE RANGE		
MO		
TU		
WE		
TH		
FR		
SA		
SU		
RADIANCE SCORE		

ABOUT THE AUTHOR

D. A. Sarac is a fiction editor, author, and playwright. Works include *Dream Big, Princess*; *The Newest Avenger*; *(Your Child) Saves the Day*; and *My Monster Friends and Me*, available from PutMeInTheStory.com and Sourcebooks. Her all-time favorite gig is being a mom to a beautiful, witty, and talented daughter. You can find her wearing a Radiant hat and alphabetizing newly learned curse words at TheEditingPen.com.

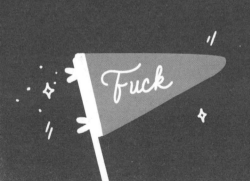